Everywhere I Am

A Prayer Journey of Health For All Women

Rochelle L. Wallace

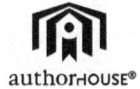
authorHOUSE®

AuthorHouse™
1663 Liberty Drive, Suite 200
Bloomington, IN 47403
www.authorhouse.com
Phone: 1-800-839-8640

First published by AuthorHouse 12/17/2008

ISBN: 978-1-4389-3183-8 (sc)

Printed in the United States of America
Bloomington, Indiana

This book is printed on acid-free paper.

All scripture quotations are taken from the New Living translation unless otherwise noted.

Dedicated To:

My Heavenly Father for being everywhere I am and beating me there every time; my mom, Betty Ellis, besides God Himself, you were the only one who could even sense that something was wrong; my aunt Pat, a twelve year breast cancer survivor; my daughter, Ameris, I love you Pumpkin, and my spiritual leaders Pastor Steve and Deidra Green, thanks for being who you are and all that you do. May God bless each of you according to His promises. I love you all!

For I am the Lord who heals you.

Exodus 15:26

Everywhere I Am

I can never escape from your Spirit!
I can never get away from your presence!
If I go up to heaven, you are there;
if I go down to the grave, you are there.

If I ride the wings of the morning,
if I dwell by the farthest oceans,
even there your hand will guide me,

Your strength will support me.
I could ask the darkness to hide me
and the light around me to become night—
but even in darkness I cannot hide from you.
To you the night shines as bright as day.
Darkness and light are the same to you.

You made all the delicate, inner parts of my body
and knit me together in my mother's womb.
Thank you for making me so wonderfully complex!
Your workmanship is marvelous—how well I know it.

Psalm 139:7-14

Contents

Introduction

This book is written for women everywhere, as all women have been, or will be impacted by the effects of breast cancer either directly or indirectly. Statistics indicate that one in eight women will be diagnosed with breast cancer. This prayer guide provides spiritual ammunition useful for the maintenance, recovery and support of your physical, emotional and spiritual health. Included as primary risk factors of breast cancer are: *(1) Being a woman and (2) Growing older.* Therefore, every woman needs ammunition in the fight against breast cancer.

Even if you are not facing the challenges of *having* breast cancer or receiving chemotherapy treatments, you will need the weaponry of prayer and the reassurance of God's presence during your life's journey. This guide offers comfort and support provided through prayer and the promises of the Word of God regardless of your location in life's journey.

You are sure to locate yourself in this journey of health, whether you are performing your monthly breast self exam, preparing for a mammogram or grieving the loss of a loved one to breast cancer, know that God is there. He is walking with you in this journey of life. Therefore, you can confidently say, *"He is.........* ***Everywhere I Am.****"*

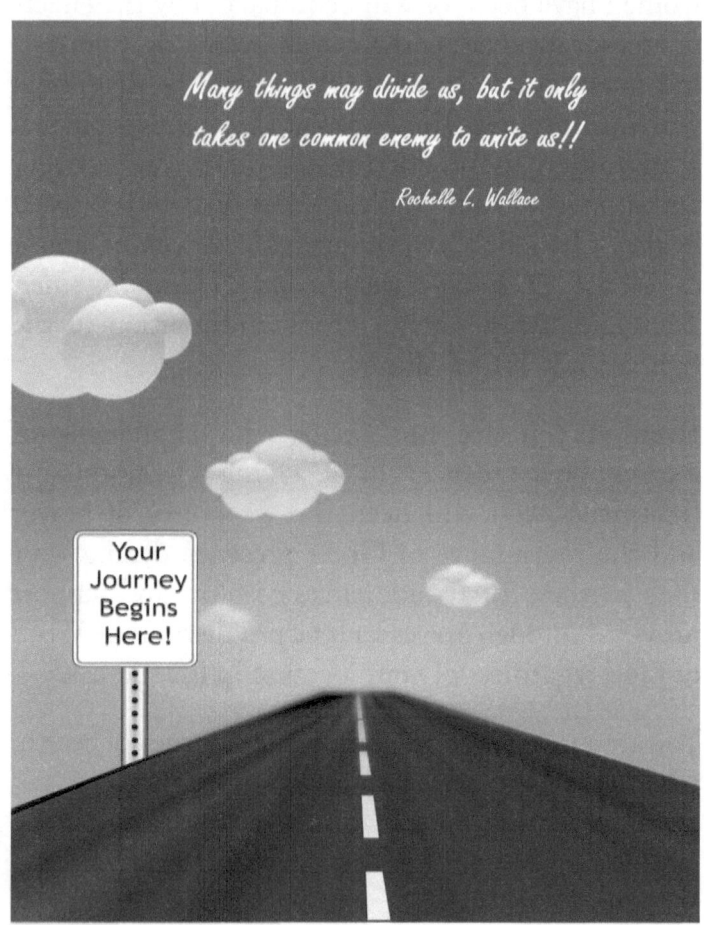

"So, what did the doctor say?" my mother asked. Oh nothing, but the usual, just to lose some weight, I jokingly responded. Little did I know 24 hours later, I would get a call that sparked the production of this booklet.

I was later called back in for a secondary reading of my mammogram. The reason for this second reading was simply stated *"they thought they saw something"*. Wow! Words can't describe the immediate floodgate of emotions that tackle you at once.

The next few days would include feelings of every imaginable variety. As I sat in the waiting room, I longed for something to help me occupy my mind, and capture my thoughts. Even with all my years of studying the word of God, I stammered for the right words and scriptures to confess and declare over the report I held in my hands.

Well, after the calming presence of the Lord engulfed me, the Lord began to encourage me through His promises. As I began to write them down, I felt the urgency to continue to pen other specific prayers, *even for the areas that I wasn't experiencing*. I soon came to realize that the Lord had sparked a mandate to help other women (in situations far more critical than what I had experienced) to communicate with Him through prayers and scriptural backing.

The following prayers are a result of my belief that believing, speaking and targeted intercession is crucial in the victory over any situation.

*For we are God's masterpiece.
He has created us anew in Christ
Jesus, so we can do the good things
he planned for us long ago.*

-Ephesians 2:10

Every Woman's Daily
Prayer for Health

Father, I thank you that I am fearfully and marvelously made. You made me and formed all my inward parts. I give you praise that every part of my being functions in the perfection to which you created it. Your word declares that you wish above all things that I prosper and be in health. Father, I agree with your word. I speak divine health and wealth over my life. My body is the temple of the living God. Help me to care for it as your dwelling place. I will not abuse, neglect, nor over indulge your temple in irresponsible acts of the flesh. I present this body to you as a living sacrifice. I trust you with my body, my spirit, my life. Thank you for keeping my body healthy and whole. Thank you for giving me wisdom, discipline, and diligence to steadfastly care for this body you have given me. I was created in your image. Help me to love and confidently say that I am the workmanship of Christ Jesus, and marvelous are thy works O Lord!

Psalm 139
III John 2
I Corinthians 6:9
Romans 12:1-2
I Thessalonians 5:23
Genesis 2:26-27
Ephesians 2:10

And let the beauty of the LORD our God be upon us: and establish thou the work of our hands upon us; yea, the work of our hands establish thou it.

-Psalm 90:17

Monthly Self-Exam Prayer

Father, God in the name of Jesus, I lift up my hands to you in total surrender. Thank you that I can lift them up without doubt and without contention or wrath. I believe your word. I have no doubt that your word is true. I meditate upon your promises of health, and I thank you for a successful exam right now in the name of Jesus. Search me and know me Lord. See if there be any wicked or unhealthy thing in me and then cleanse and remove it from me Lord. I ask you according to your word, Lord, teach my hands to war and my fingers to fight. I claim victory and a good report from this exam in the name of Jesus.

See your local breast health specialist for the latest in breast self exam techniques.

Psalm 144:1
Philippians 4:6
I Tim. 2:8
Joshua 1:8

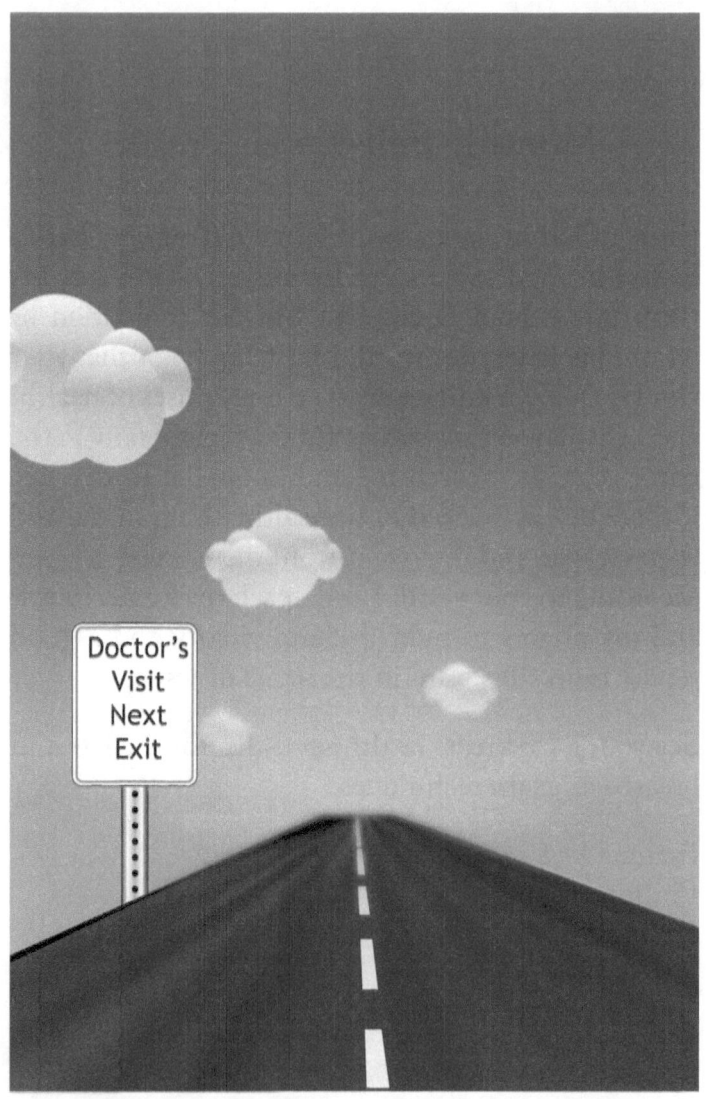

Pre-Mammogram Prayers

The Waiting Room Prayer
Awaiting Test Results Prayer

Don't worry about anything; instead, pray about everything. Tell God what you need, and thank him for all He has done. Then you will experience God's peace, which exceeds anything we can understand. His peace will guard your hearts and minds as you live in Christ Jesus.

– Phillipians 4:6-7

Pre-Mammogram Prayer
"Waiting Room Prayer"

Father, I thank you that my body is the temple of the Living God. Therefore, because you live in me, no ungodly nor unholy thing can dwell within this body. Father, I thank you that the report of the Lord reigns over my life. Your report says that I am already healed. Therefore, I expect a report of health from my mammogram. I thank you that there is no illegal formation of clusters nor abnormal cellular activity in my body. Any and all signs of abnormal density are cursed to the roots, and I decree that my breasts are healthy. My lymph nodes and glands are healthy. I thank you for a pain-free testing and a clear and accurate reading that reflects your report of good health. I decree that my cellular tissue lines up to that which you created it and my body belongs to you, spirit, soul, and body. I am not afraid! I am not afraid! I am not afraid! Father, you have not given me a spirit of fear, but one of love, power and a sound mind. By the same power that raised Jesus from the dead, I decree a good report…. NOW!!!

In the name of Jesus, the word of God says that you made me in your image. You fashioned even my very inward parts. Right now in the name of Jesus I decree that anything that you by your divine wisdom did not place or ordain to live in my body must dissipate and vacate my body, now! I plead the protection of the blood of Jesus. Thank you for a mammogram (ultrasound) report that reads clear and healthy. Now Father, I ask you to search me, my breasts, my biopsy and my heart. See if there be any wicked or unhealthy thing in me. I ask you to take it out Lord, that I may live!!

I Cor. 6:19
Psalm 139:13
Genesis 1:26
Psalm 139:23&24
Psalm 139:16
Proverbs 20:27

And now, dear brothers and sisters, one final thing. Fix your thoughts on what is true, and honorable, and right, and pure, and lovely, and admirable. Think about things that are excellent and worthy of praise.

— Philippians 4:8

Pre-Mammogram Results Prayer
Awaiting Test Results Prayer

I thank you for the good report from my mammogram *(or other tests)*. According to Jeremiah 29:11, you already have plans for me, good plans. Your word says that those plans include an expected end for me. Father, I expect the resulting end of my mammogram to give a good report. I expect an accurate report of health, with no signs of discrepancies nor abnormalities. Father, my heart is indicting a good matter and I decree the end from the beginning. God is my refuge and my strength, therefore, my heart will not fear. Right now Lord, I cast the whole of any care upon you, because I know that you care for me. Whatsoever things are lovely, pure and of a good report, I choose to meditate on them. Thank you Father for the good report!

Isaiah 26:3
Isaiah 53:1
Jeremiah 29:11
Psalm 18:23
Psalm 45:1
Psalm 46:1-2
Psalm 46:10
Job 22:28
Philippians 4:8
I Peter 5:7

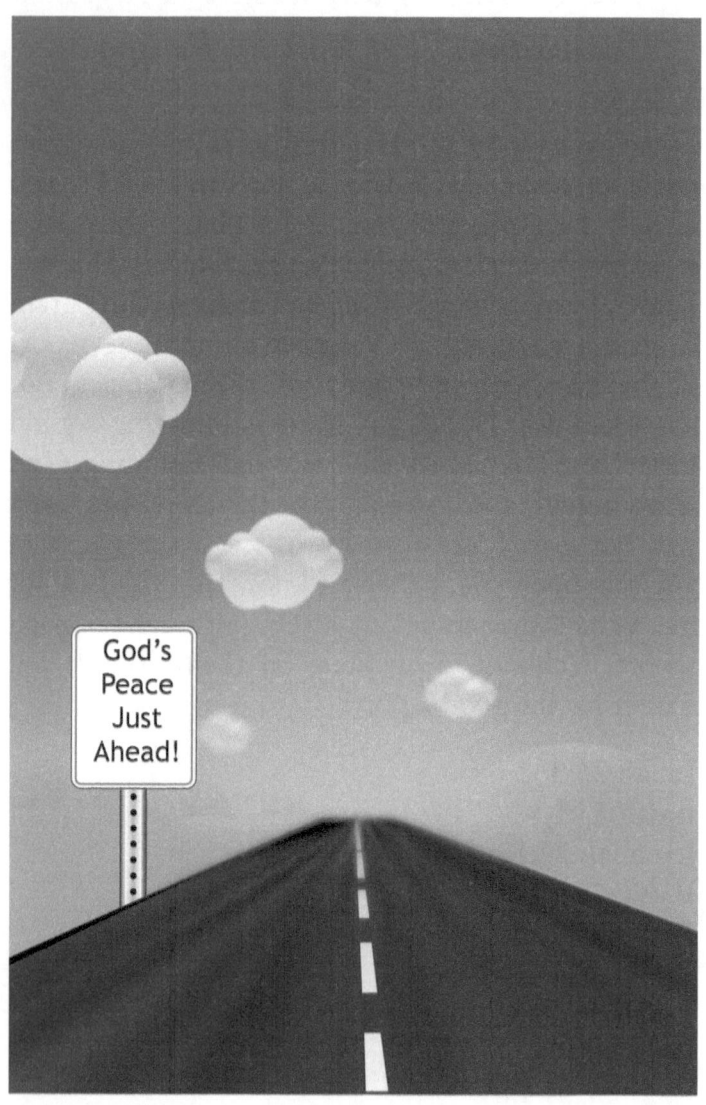

Post-Mammogram Prayers

Prayer of Thanksgiving
When Additional Testing is Needed Prayer

You guide me with your counsel,
leading me to a glorious destiny.

– Psalm 73:24

Prayer of Thanksgiving

Thank you Lord! Thank you that you have again redeemed my life from destruction! As a bird from the snare of the fowler, You have allowed me to escape and my soul cries hallelujah! Thank you Lord for saving me! As your word declares, yes Lord, I will sing of your mercies forever! With *my* mouth I will tell everyone of your faithfulness. I bless you now and rejoice for the many that will come to know you as a result of this awesome testimony of healing and deliverance!

Psalm 86:13
Psalm 89:1
Psalm 91:3
Psalm 124:7
Lamentations 3:57-58
Rev. 12:11

You will keep in perfect peace all who trust in you, all whose thoughts are fixed on you!

- Isaiah 26:3

When Additional Screening Is Needed Prayer

No weapon formed against me shall prosper. Lord your word states that I am already healed by the stripes of Jesus. You said let every word of God be established by two or three witnesses. Thank you Father that this secondary reading serves only to confirm your report of health over my life! Thank you for your peace! I will have rest and sleep just as your word declares! Yet will I praise you, because I know that my Redeemer lives.

Reference Scriptures:
Luke 18:1-7
Isaiah 26:3
Job 19:25
Psalm 3:4-5
Isaiah 54:17
Isaiah 59:16
Habakkuk 3:17-19

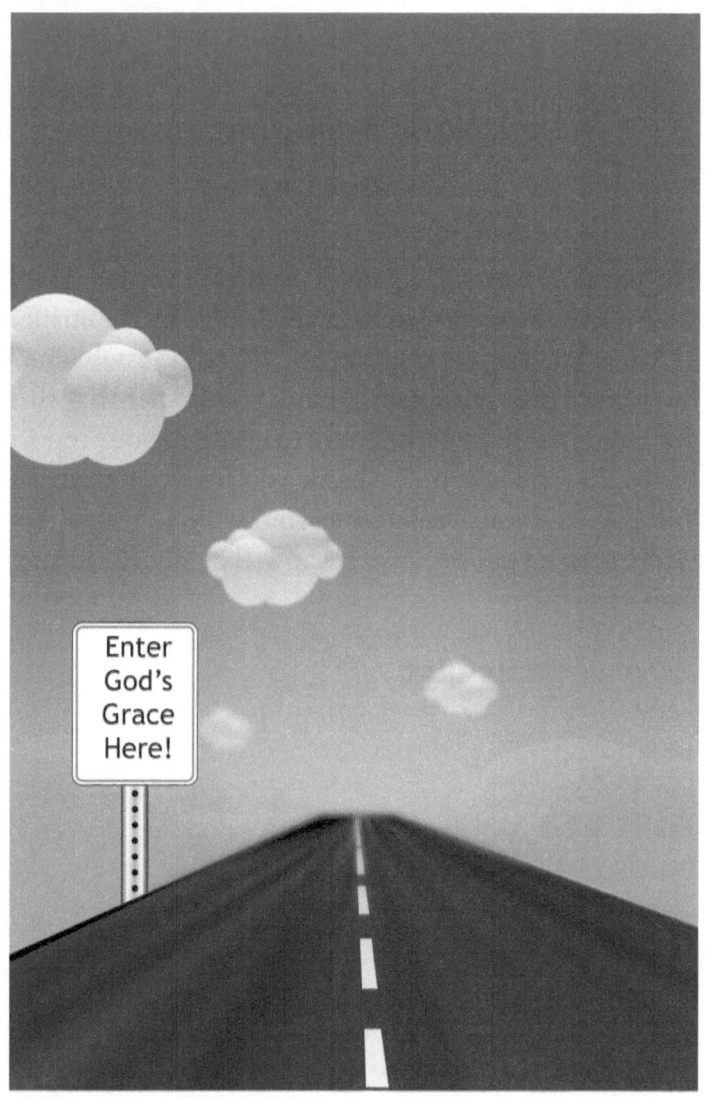

Treatment Prayers

Pre-Chemotherapy/Radiation Prayer
Day of Treatment Prayer
Treatment Prayer
Post-Treatment Thanksgiving Prayer

*And we know that God causes
everything to work together for the good
of those who love God and are called
according to his purpose for them.*

– Romans 8:28

Pre-Chemotherapy/Radiation Prayer

Father, I thank you for going before me. Just as it was with Elijah at the brook of Cherith, I thank you that the blessed gift of healing has already been prepared and awaits me. Thank you that as I go for treatment, healing is already mine. Each round of therapy/treatment is a step toward that ordained place. I release the hold and give you free course and reign within these treatments. O Lord, according to Thy loving-kindness, let nausea be removed from me. According to your word, the very hairs of my head are numbered. Not one hair will fall from my head without your knowledge, and you make all things beautiful in its time! Your word declares that a fire goes before you to burn up all your enemies. Cancer and sickness are enemies to your word and promise of health. Thru the technological advancements that you have allowed and ordained, burn out the cancerous cells that may have invaded this body! Thank you for your promise to be with me, even when I go thru the fire! I will fear no evil, for Thou art with me.

Isaiah 43:2
Psalm 97:3
Matthew 10:28-31

Everyone tried to touch him, because healing power went out from him, and he healed everyone.

-Luke 6:19

Day of Treatment Prayer

Surely, there is an end, and my expectation shall not be cut off! (Proverbs 23:18) You promised to never leave me, nor forsake me. Thank you that you have already anointed my head with oil. My cup runneth over. Thank you that your healing virtue still flows and today it reaches me! Thank you that healing is the children's bread. Right now I partake in this meal of health and deliverance. I agree with your word and decree that these treatments are working together for my good.

Isaiah 54:17
Hebrews 13:5
Proverbs 23:18
Psalm 143:11
Romans 8:28

Christ in you, the hope of glory!!

— Colossians 1:27 (KJV)

Chemotherapy / Radiation Treatment Prayer

Father, I thank you that you are everywhere I am. When I go through the fire you are there with me. Your word declares that a fire goes before me and burns up any and everything that adversely affects my health or that has lodged within my body. I command that there be no abnormal growth, reproduction, or assembly of cells in my body. Any foreign body or malignancy is cursed to the root. I command it by the power and authority of the blood of Jesus to dry up and be removed from my body in the name of Jesus! All consuming fire, burn away every cancerous cell by your fire! I thank you that I am redeemed from the curse of the law and that there are no adverse side effects from treatment. You have numbered the very hairs of my head, and hair is symbolic of the glory. Because your glory engulfs me as your manifested presence, I thank you that you establish and restore your glory in me. I will not acquire nor receive unnecessary and unwarranted warfare as a result of treatment. I am More Than A Conqueror. I can do all things through Christ, who gives me strength. I am beloved of God. You promised never to leave nor forsake me and because You are my Shepherd, I will fear no evil; Your rod and Your staff comfort me. I know that this light affliction is only working a far more exceeding weight of glory, and I shall not die, but live and declare the works of the Lord!

Hebrews 12:29
John 15:15
Philippians 4:13
Psalm 23
Psalm 97:3
Psalm 118:13
Romans 8:36-37
Galatians 3:13

*Let all that I am praise the L*ORD*;*
may I never forget the good things
he does for me. He forgives all my
sins and heals all my diseases.

- Psalm 103:1-3

Post Treatment Prayer
of Thanksgiving

Thank you for the success of the treatment. Thank You Lord for the confirming good report that testifies of Your miraculous power in my body. I praise you knowing that not only were my treatments successful, but according to Nahum 1:9, affliction will not arise in my body again; no, not another time. Thank you that your healing virtue is at work and flowing through my body now in the name of Jesus. My stamina, strength, health and total capacity is restored in the name of Jesus. According to the promise of your word, everything that the cankerworm hath stolen from me must be restored. I praise you now for this awesome restoration, for you have dealt wondrously with me!

Joel 2:25
Nahum 1:9
Luke 1:35
Luke 6:19
I Corinthians 15:57
II Corinthians 2:14

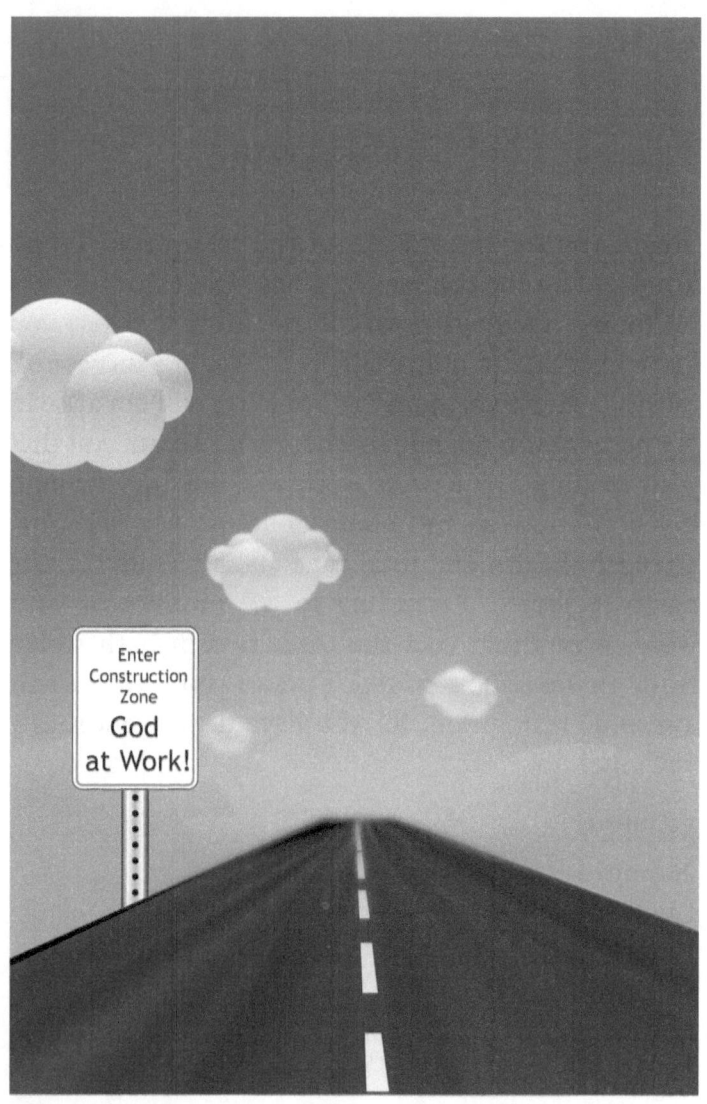

Surgical Prayers

Pre-Surgical Prayer
Post-Surgical Prayer
Remission and Healing Prayer
Post-Treatment Prayer

By his divine power, God has given us everything we need for living a godly life. We have received all of this by coming to know him, the one who called us to himself by means of his marvelous glory and excellence.

- II Peter 1:3

Pre-Surgical Prayer

Blessed be the Lord that teaches our hands to war and our fingers to fight. I ask you Father to guide the surgeon's hands as he engages into this warfare on my behalf. Show him/her the path of life for me. Reveal what is necessary to sustain my life. Anoint his/her eyes with eye salve from heaven that they may see every natural defect or potential threat as well as any hidden hindrances to my health. I put my trust in you because you are the Great Physician. My life is in your hand and I trust you because you are the true lifegiver. You are the resurrection and the life! Your word is life and brings continual healing to me. Therefore, Father allow your sharp, quick, and powerful word to perform this surgery on my behalf, even before the surgeon begins. As your word cuts and divides, Lord let it release healing to all my inward parts.

Psalm 16:10-11
Psalm 144:1
Jeremiah 33:3
John 11:25
John 14:6

Then your salvation will come like the dawn, and <u>your wounds will quickly heal.</u> Your godliness will lead you forward, and the glory of the LORD will protect you from behind.

— Isaiah 58:8

Post-Surgical Prayer

Thank you for a successful surgery! I am fearfully and wonderfully made. Father, I thank you for the money and the favor that covers everything that makes for my peace. This includes reconstruction, clothing, and anything for my overall support. Jehovah Rophe', thank you for a speedy and thorough recovery. I will not experience unnecessary pains nor discomfort within my body. I decree that supernatural strength is infused within my body in the name of Jesus and I am in every way whole; spirit, soul and body. Thank you for causing me to arise in total health even as the Son of Righteousness arises with healing in His wings!!!

Psalm 139
Proverbs 3:3
Isaiah 60:1
I Thessalonians 5:23

Give thanks to the Lord*, for He is good! His faithful love endures forever. Give thanks to the God of gods. His faithful love endures forever. Give thanks to the Lord of lords. His faithful love endures forever. Give thanks to Him who alone does mighty miracles. His faithful love endures forever.*

- Psalm 136:1-4

Prayer for Remission/Healing

I will love thee O my God. I will praise thee because you have heard my cry. You have answered my prayers. By your stripes, I am walking in complete, victorious healing. Since You were wounded and bruised for my transgressions and iniquities, I am able to walk free from the curse of sickness and disease. Blessed be the Lord who this day hath loaded me with the benefit of healing and healed my body of all diseases. Thank you that cancer will not rise again within this body. I thank you for healing this body and saving me from death. I will praise you Lord for your loving-kindness and tender mercies toward me. Surely, it was only because your mercy that I have been spared. Thus, I will magnify you in this body in the name of Jesus!! Now Lord even as Paul, I dwell not on the things which are behind me, but I continue to press on toward the prize and my High call from You, my Lord, Jesus Christ.

Psalm 103:1-3
Jeremiah 33:3
Lamentations 3:22
I Corinthians 6:19
Philippians 3:14

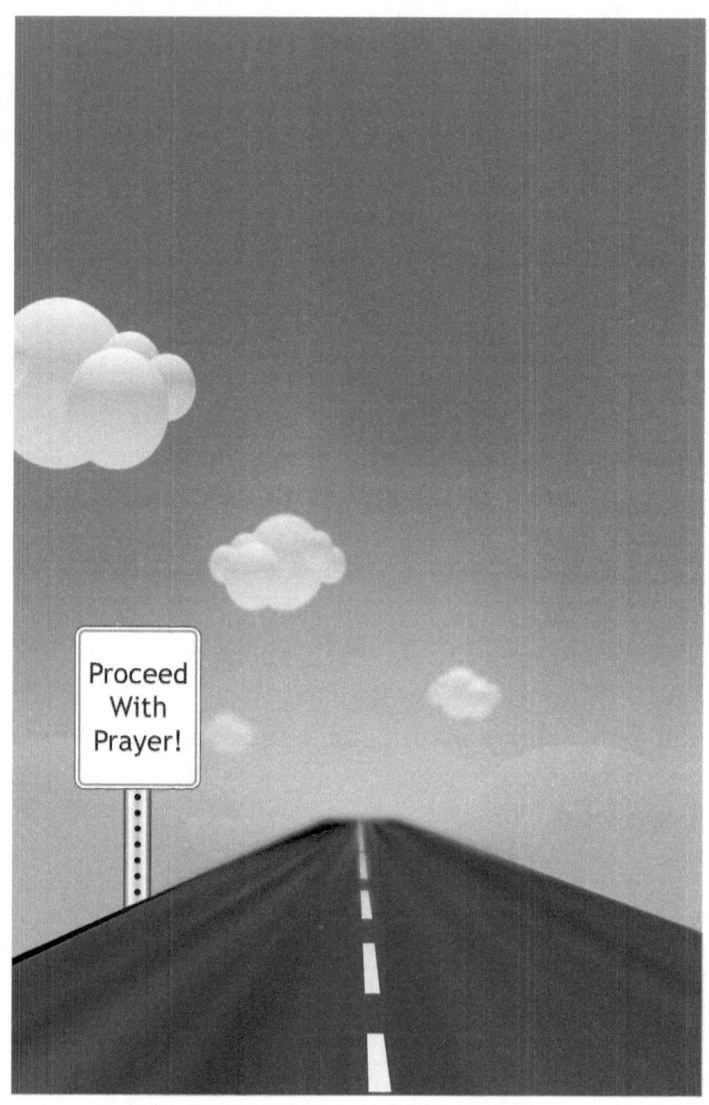

Specialty Prayers

Prayer for Families of Cancer Patients
Prayer for Grieving Families
Prayer for Physicians,
Nurses and Other Medical Staff
Prayer For a Cure
Prayer For Men Facing Breast Cancer

A person standing alone can be attacked and defeated, but two can stand back-to-back and conquer. Three are even better, for a triple-braided cord is not easily broken.

– Ecclesiastes 4:12

Prayer for Families of Breast Cancer Patients

Father, I pray for the _____ family. I pray that you have already blessed them with all things that pertain to life and godliness. I pray for increased sensitivity to one another's needs during this time. Thank you that all of their needs are met physically, spiritually, financially, and emotionally. Father remind them that a threefold cord is not easily broken. Therefore, with You, the patient, and the family combined it means total defeat over the enemy is assured in this fight. Now thanks be to God who has given them the victory through Christ Jesus. May the _____ family begin to raise up a new standard of praise that will still the enemy as they reclaim their health's redemption through Christ Jesus. May they walk together in love, unity and agreement, causing their faith in you to be activated in their behalf.

Amos 3:3
Philippians 4:19
Isaiah 59:19
Psalm 8
Galatians 5:6

Then you will experience God's peace,
which exceeds anything we can understand.
His peace will guard your hearts and
minds as you live in Christ Jesus.

– Philippians 4:7

Grieving Families

You are the God of peace and comfort. I will not charge God foolishly. Thou art holy O Lord. I pray that your peace engulfs the _____ family and overshadows them with your love. Holy Spirit rain down upon them and wrap them in your arms of consolation. Jehovah Shalom grant them peace as you promised Your beloved. I pray according to your word that The Comforter abides in the _____ home, and shall ease their hearts and minds.

Psalm 3
Psalm 22
Isaiah 26:3
John 14:1
John 14:16
I Thessalonians 4:13

The LORD directs the steps of the godly.
He delights in every detail of their lives.

– Psalm 37:23

For by wise counsel you can wage
your war, and in an abundance of
counselors there is victory and safety.

- Proverbs 24:6 (Amplified Version)

Prayer for Physicians, Nurses, Other Medical Staff

Lord, order my steps. Lead me to the physician and staff that is best for me and will provide the treatment needed for my best results. Let the doctor I receive be the best for my case and treatment. May the nurses and staff surrounding and attending me be God sent and ordained to best aid in my healing and recovery. May the supporting staff compliment the physician and service provided to me. I pray for them and the things that make for their peace as well. Regardless of my circumstances I pray that you bless them and keep them, make your face to shine upon them and give them peace. I pray that they will receive and offer Godly counsel for my good and safety. Father as wise professionals of medicine, let them dig deep for wise counsel for my good health.

Numbers 6:24
Psalm 73:24
Proverbs 3:6
Proverbs 9:9-10
Proverbs 11:14
Proverbs 15:22
Proverbs 20:18

*For the time is coming when everything
that is covered will be revealed, and all
that is secret will be made known to all.*

— Matthew 10:26

Prayer for a Cure

Father there have been many human efforts within the fight of breast cancer, but I know that your word says that the weapons of our warfare are not carnal, but they are mighty thru God to the pulling down of strongholds. This ungodly disease has plagued our land long enough and we pray for an intervention from heaven. Just as in days of old we ask that the plague be stayed. According to II Chronicles, we ask that you heal our land as we humble ourselves before You . We seek your face for the answer for the cure. Father, grant knowledge and witty inventions to researchers, physicians, patients, and loved ones that will result in comfort, relief, and healing to those suffering from this disease. Grant medical, scientific, and holistic knowledge that will not be commercialized to stay the hand of the enemy and end the sting of breast cancer forever! Father reveal Your hidden wisdom for the cure. I ask you to bring from darkness to the light wisdom for prevention, treatment and cures that are hidden.

II Chronicles 7:14
Ezekiel 22:30
Proverbs 8:12
I Corinthians 2:7
I Corinthians 4:5
II Corinthians 10:3-6

*Behold, I have indelibly imprinted
(tattooed a picture of) you on the
palm of each of My hands; your
walls are continually before Me.*

- Isaiah 49:16 (Amplified Version)

Men Facing Breast Cancer

Father, I bind fear, timidity, embarrassment, and pride. Thank you that I am not forgotten. You have engraved me in the palm of your hand and I am the apple of your eye. Surely goodness and mercy follows me, and I am never alone. Your healing virtue flows to me and thru me. You are not a respecter of persons. Thank you that I am a whole man of God; spirit, soul and body, and I walk in total healing and victory!

Psalm 23
Proverbs 16:18
Zechariah 2:8
Acts 10:34
I Thessalonians 5:23
II Timothy 1:7

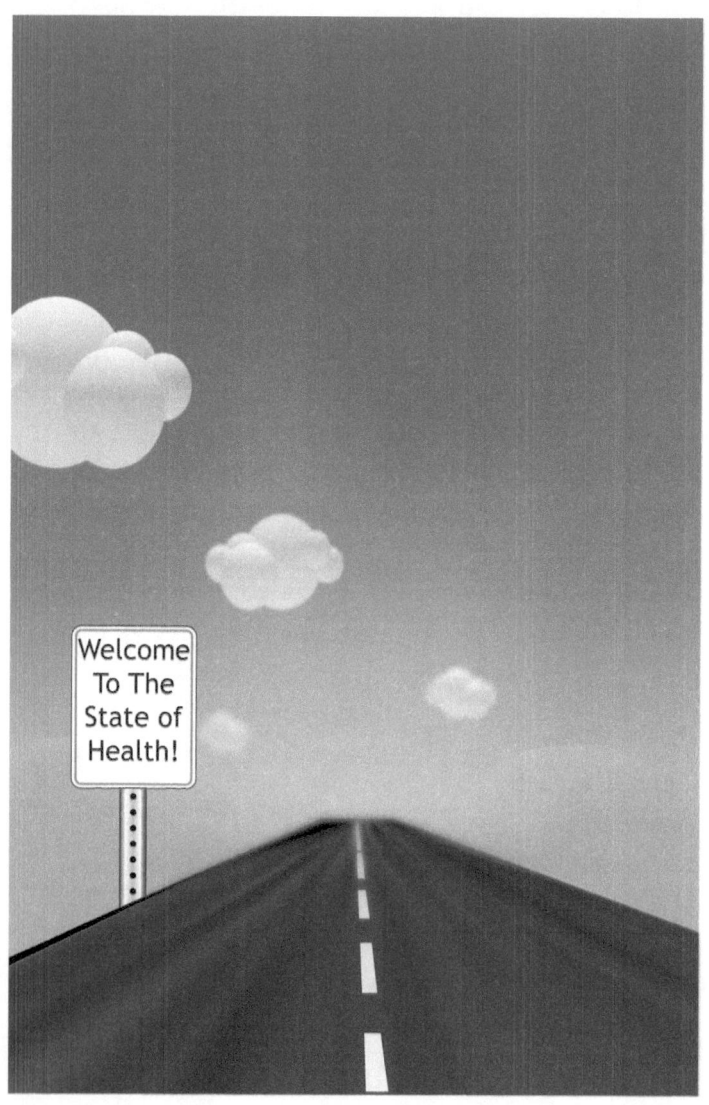

By the grace of God my testing came back showing no signs or traces of _anything_ on the second reading and ultrasound.

The sheer anxiety and feelings of aloneness sparked a fire of prayer and study of the scriptures for biblical promises specifically designed for each stage in a woman's health journey. This includes those walking in health as well as those undergoing treatment or in remission.

Although this is the concluding page of the prayer booklet, it was actually completed first. In fact, the first night I began writing, I began to pen this page. This was my concluding statement, even prior to a repeat mammogram, ultrasound, or additional testing. Why or how would God allow me to write this booklet? I believe that true, heartfelt, intercessory prayer comes best when you pray for someone else (just as if it was you).

You may be wondering how I knew the outcome. How were you able to be so confident, you may ask? According to the word of God, you can declare the end from the beginning. You can decree a thing and it shall come to pass. (Job 22:28-30) That verse continues by saying that others can be delivered by the cleanness of your own hands. By completing the prayers within this book, I somehow feel the weight of the blood, of other women's lives, has been washed from my hands.

The wasted time of fear in the waiting room doesn't have to plague another woman, as we now have a *"Waiting Room Prayer"*. As a result of reading through this healing journey, others can now be spared the frustration of frantically searching for scriptures while waiting on test results and may now be encouraged by God's promises for the situations and places they may walk. May you find rest in His peace and confidence in knowing that He is…….

Everywhere You Are!!

Topical Listing of Scriptures

Meditation
Philippians 4:6
Joshua 1:8
Isaiah 26:3
Psalm 139:23-24
I Cor. 6:19
Psalm 45:1

Mercy
Psalm 86:13
Psalm 89:1
Lamentations 3:22

Prayer
II Chronicles 7:14
Psalm 22:24
Isaiah 59:16
Jeremiah 33:3
Ezekiel 22:30
Luke 18:1-7

Presence of the Lord
Isaiah 43:2
Psalm 23:4
Hebrews 13:5

Topical Listing of Scriptures

Body
Psalm 139:14
III John 2
I Corinthians 6:19
Romans 12:1-2
I Thessalonians 5:23
Genesis 1:26-27
Ephesians 2:10

Counsel
Psalm 73:24
Proverbs 11:14
Proverbs 15:22

Fear
Psalm 46:1-2
II Timothy 1:7
Matthew 10:28-30

Hands
Psalm 144:1
I Tim. 2:8

Life
John 11:25
John 14:6
Psalm 16:10-11

Topical Listing of Scriptures

The Lord's Plan/Report
Isaiah 53:1
Jeremiah 29:11
Proverbs 23:18

Victory
I Corinthians 15:57
II Corinthians 2:14

Warfare/Defense
Psalm 8:2
Proverbs 20:18
Isaiah 54:17
Isaiah 59:19
II Corinthians 10:3-6

Rest In the Lord
Psalm 3:4-5
Psalm 46:10
Philippians 4:8
I Peter 5:7
Job 19:25
John 14:1
John 14:16

Restoration
Joel 2:25
Nahum 1:9